Nurturing Generations: A Guide to Women's Reproductive Health

Table of Contents

Introduction

In the intricate tapestry of life, the health and well-being of women hold a profound significance. Women are not just the bearers of generations but also the architects of societies. Their physical and reproductive health is the cornerstone upon which societies are built, yet it remains one of the most misunderstood and often misrepresented aspects of human existence.

As we embark on this journey through the pages of "Nurturing Generations: A Guide to Women's Reproductive Health," we are venturing into a world that has long been obscured by myths, shrouded in taboos, and plagued by misinformation. This book stands as a beacon of knowledge, illuminating the path to understanding and empowerment for women of all ages and backgrounds, across the globe.

The need for such a comprehensive guide has never been more evident. In a world that is constantly evolving, where cultures and traditions intermingle, where healthcare systems vary greatly, and where the digital age offers both a wealth of information and a sea of misinformation, women must navigate the labyrinth of reproductive health with clarity and confidence.

From the very inception of this project, it became abundantly clear that the importance of women's reproductive health transcends geographical boundaries, cultural norms, and socioeconomic disparities. Whether in the bustling urban centers of developed nations or the remote villages of the developing world, women share a common thread – the need for accurate information, compassionate care, and the empowerment to make informed choices about their own bodies.

In the pages that follow, we will embark on a holistic exploration of women's reproductive health, spanning the entire spectrum of a woman's life – from the innocent days of childhood to the wisdom of old age. We will delve into the mysteries of puberty, the challenges of the reproductive years, the transformative journey of pregnancy and motherhood, the sometimes perplexing transition through perimenopause and menopause, and the nuanced aspects of reproductive health in later life.

This book does not merely provide information; it serves as a trusted companion, a confidante, and a guide. It dispels myths and misconceptions, replacing them with evidence-based knowledge. It offers practical advice and accessible remedies, embracing the diversity of cultures and healthcare systems around the world.

Moreover, it acknowledges that women's reproductive health is not a solitary journey but a collective one. It pays tribute to the stories of countless women who have faced challenges, overcome obstacles, and emerged stronger. Their voices resonate throughout these pages, reminding us of the resilience and strength that define the essence of womanhood.

As we embark on this voyage, we extend an invitation to women of all ages and backgrounds, to healthcare professionals and advocates, and to anyone who seeks a deeper understanding of women's reproductive health. Together, we shall embark on a journey of empowerment, where knowledge dispels fear, where compassion replaces stigma, and where the well-being of women becomes the cornerstone upon which healthier, happier societies are built.

Welcome to "Nurturing Generations: A Guide to Women's Reproductive Health." Your journey towards empowerment and enlightenment begins here.

Chapter 1: Foundations of Reproductive Health

In the opening chapter of "Nurturing Generations: A Guide to Women's Reproductive Health," we embark on a journey to establish a solid foundation of knowledge. This foundation is crucial because understanding the intricacies of reproductive health is the first step towards making informed decisions, dispelling myths, and nurturing holistic wellness throughout a woman's life.

At its core, reproductive health encompasses the physical, mental, and social well-being related to the reproductive system. It goes beyond the absence of disease or dysfunction; it embraces the concept of wellness, which implies a state of optimal health. Reproductive health acknowledges that a woman's well-being is deeply intertwined with her reproductive system, and it emphasizes the importance of both maintaining this system's health and addressing any issues that may arise.

Understanding reproductive health also involves recognizing that it's not solely about fertility or pregnancy. It encompasses the entire life span of a woman, from her earliest days to the golden years of her life. This holistic approach recognizes that every stage of life presents unique challenges and opportunities for well-being, making it essential to address reproductive health comprehensively.

<u>Myths vs. Facts: Common Misconceptions</u>

One of the greatest obstacles to achieving reproductive health is the prevalence of myths and misconceptions. These myths often stem from cultural beliefs, misinformation, or a lack of comprehensive education. In this section, we'll dissect some common myths and replace them with evidence-based facts:

Myth 1: Women should have a menstrual cycle of exactly 28 days

Fact: The menstrual cycle varies among individuals and can range from 21 to 35 days. Irregularities are common and can be influenced by various factors, including stress, diet, and hormonal changes.

Myth 2: Birth control methods always lead to infertility

Fact: Most modern birth control methods are reversible, and fertility usually returns once the method is discontinued. However, individual responses can vary.

Myth 3: Women can't get pregnant while breastfeeding

Fact: While breastfeeding can suppress ovulation, it is not a foolproof method of contraception. It's essential to use appropriate birth control if avoiding pregnancy is the goal.

Myth 4: You can't get a sexually transmitted infection (STI) from oral sex

Fact: STIs can be transmitted through oral sex. It's crucial to practice safe sex, including the use of barriers like dental dams or condoms.

The Life Stages of Women

Understanding women's reproductive health requires recognizing the distinct stages that every woman experiences during her lifetime. These stages, though unique in their challenges and characteristics, are interconnected and lay the foundation for a woman's overall reproductive well-being.

Childhood: The journey begins in childhood, where education about one's body is paramount. Girls should be taught about the basics of anatomy, menstruation, and hygiene. This knowledge sets the stage for a healthier transition into adolescence.

Adolescence: Puberty marks the transition to adolescence, a stage characterized by rapid physical and emotional changes. Menarche, the first menstrual period, typically occurs during this time. Girls need support and accurate information to navigate these changes confidently.

Reproductive Years: This phase covers the years of fertility and childbearing. It involves understanding the menstrual cycle, contraception, family planning, and addressing common gynecological conditions like menstrual disorders and infections.

Pregnancy and Motherhood: Pregnancy is a transformative journey that requires careful attention to both physical and emotional well-being. This stage involves prenatal care, labor and delivery, postpartum care, and breastfeeding.

Per menopause and Menopause: As women approach middle age, per menopause heralds the transition to menopause. This phase can be marked by hormonal changes and symptoms like hot flashes and mood swings. Understanding and managing these changes is crucial.

Golden Years of Reproductive Health: Beyond menopause, a woman enters the golden years. Reproductive health during this phase involves maintaining bone health, pelvic health, and addressing any concerns related to intimacy and sexual health.

The Importance of Holistic Wellness

Holistic wellness acknowledges that a woman's reproductive health is not isolated but interconnected with her overall well-being. It recognizes that physical, mental, and social aspects of health are intertwined and must be nurtured together.

Physical Wellness: This aspect encompasses maintaining a healthy lifestyle through proper nutrition, regular exercise, and adequate sleep. It also involves regular gynecological check-ups and screenings to detect and address potential issues.

Mental Wellness: Emotional and mental health are equally vital. Stress management, self-care, and seeking support when needed are essential components of mental well-being. Reproductive health can be influenced by mental health, and vice versa.

Social Wellness: A woman's social environment, relationships, and access to healthcare play a significant role in her reproductive health. Access to education, healthcare services, and support networks are crucial factors in achieving holistic wellness.

Chapter 2: Childhood and Adolescence

In the critical stage of childhood and adolescence, understanding and nurturing reproductive health is paramount. This chapter in "Nurturing Generations: A Guide to Women's Reproductive Health" delves deeply into the experiences of girls during this transformative period, addressing the physical, emotional, and educational aspects that form the foundation of lifelong reproductive well-being.

<u>Understanding Puberty</u>

Puberty is a phase of rapid physical and emotional development that marks the transition from childhood to adolescence. It's a unique and sometimes challenging period for girls, as their bodies undergo profound changes. Understanding these changes is crucial, as it sets the stage for a healthy and informed journey through adolescence and beyond.

Physical Changes: Puberty brings physical transformations, including breast development, the growth of body hair, and the onset of menstruation. These changes are driven by hormonal shifts, particularly the increase in estrogen.

Emotional Changes: Alongside physical changes, girls may experience emotional fluctuations. Hormones can influence mood swings, and girls may navigate feelings of self-consciousness and self-identity.

Educational Component: Schools and parents play a significant role in providing comprehensive sex education. This education should cover both the biological aspects of puberty and emotional well-being, helping girls embrace these changes confidently.

Myths vs. Facts: Dispelling Misconceptions

Puberty often comes with its share of myths and misconceptions. Dispelling these myths with accurate information is crucial for girls' well-being.

Myth 1: Menstruation is dirty or impure.

Fact: Menstruation is a natural biological process and not unclean. Girls should be taught proper hygiene practices during menstruation.

Myth 2: You can't get pregnant during your first period.

Fact: While the chances are lower, it's still possible to get pregnant during the first few menstrual cycles.

Myth 3: Using tampons can break the hymen.

Fact: Tampons do not necessarily break the hymen. The hymen can have various shapes and may not completely cover the vaginal opening.

Myth 4: Period pain is normal and doesn't need medical attention.

Fact: While some discomfort can be normal, severe period pain may indicate underlying issues that require medical evaluation.

Menstrual Health Education

Menstrual health education is a fundamental component of reproductive health knowledge for girls. It encompasses various aspects:

Menstrual Cycle: Girls should understand the menstrual cycle, including the phases of menstruation, ovulation, and hormonal changes.

Hygiene and Management: Proper hygiene practices and menstrual product options (e.g., pads, tampons, and menstrual cups) should be discussed. Girls should be encouraged to choose what suits them best.

Pain and Discomfort: Educating girls about common menstrual symptoms like cramps and providing tips for managing them empowers them to handle their periods comfortably.

Emotional Well-being: Girls should be taught that emotional changes during their menstrual cycle are normal. Open conversations about mood swings and emotional well-being help reduce stigma.

<u>Nutritional Needs for Girls</u>

Nutrition plays a pivotal role in a girl's physical development during puberty. Ensuring adequate nutrient intake is vital to support growth and hormonal changes:

Calcium and Vitamin D: These are essential for bone health, especially during puberty when bones grow rapidly.

Iron: Girls need more iron during menstruation to replace the blood they lose. Iron-rich foods like lean meats, beans, and leafy greens are crucial.

Fiber and Hydration: A diet rich in fiber and proper hydration helps manage constipation, a common issue during menstruation.

Balanced Diet: Encourage girls to maintain a balanced diet with a variety of fruits, vegetables, grains, and protein sources.

<u>Emotional Well-being</u>

Emotional well-being during adolescence is as important as physical health. Puberty can be emotionally challenging, and girls need support:

Peer Pressure and Self-Esteem: Adolescence often involves peer pressure. Girls should learn to build self-esteem and assertiveness to make healthy choices.

Body Image and Self-acceptance: Addressing body image issues is crucial. Girls should be encouraged to embrace their changing bodies and develop a positive self-image.

Stress Management: Coping with academic and social pressures is part of adolescence. Teaching stress management techniques can help girls navigate these challenges.

Open Communication: Creating a safe space for open communication is vital. Girls should feel comfortable discussing their concerns, fears, and questions about puberty and their bodies.

This Chapter focuses on the crucial period of childhood and adolescence, where girls embark on their journey through puberty. Understanding the physical and emotional changes, dispelling myths, providing menstrual health education, addressing nutritional needs, and nurturing emotional well-being are essential elements in laying a strong foundation for reproductive health. By empowering girls with knowledge and support during this phase, we equip them to make informed decisions and embrace their reproductive well-being with confidence and resilience.

Chapter 3: The Reproductive Years

In the journey through "Nurturing Generations: A Guide to Women's Reproductive Health," we arrive at the pivotal chapter focused on the reproductive years. This phase encompasses a substantial portion of a woman's life, from the onset of menstruation to the years leading up to menopause. It's a period marked by significant physiological changes, the potential for childbearing, and the importance of informed choices regarding reproductive health.

<u>Menstrual Cycle and Ovulation</u>

Understanding the Menstrual Cycle:

The menstrual cycle is a complex and rhythmic process that occurs in most women of reproductive age. It typically lasts 21 to 35 days, although individual variations are common. The menstrual cycle can be divided into several phases:

1. Menstruation: The cycle begins with menstruation, during which the uterine lining sheds. This phase typically lasts 3 to 7 days.

2. Follicular Phase: Following menstruation, the body enters the follicular phase. During this time, the pituitary gland

releases follicle-stimulating hormone (FSH), which stimulates the ovaries to produce follicles.

3. Ovulation: Ovulation is a crucial event in the menstrual cycle. It occurs when a mature egg is released from an ovarian follicle, typically around the midpoint of the cycle. Ovulation is triggered by a surge in luteinizing hormone (LH). Understanding when ovulation occurs is vital for both family planning and fertility.

4. Luteal Phase: After ovulation, the body enters the luteal phase. During this phase, the ruptured follicle transforms into a structure called the corpus luteum, which produces progesterone. Progesterone prepares the uterine lining for a potential pregnancy.

5. Potential Pregnancy: If fertilization occurs, the fertilized egg travels to the uterus and implants into the uterine lining. If not, the corpus luteum breaks down, progesterone levels drop, and menstruation begins again, marking the start of a new cycle.

Understanding the menstrual cycle is fundamental to reproductive health, as it provides valuable insights into fertility, contraception, and overall gynecological well-being.

<u>Contraception and Family Planning</u>

Contraception Options:

The reproductive years are a prime time for considering family planning and contraception. There are numerous contraception options available to women, each with its benefits and considerations:

1. Hormonal Methods: These include birth control pills, patches, and hormonal intrauterine devices (IUDs). They work by altering hormone levels to prevent pregnancy.

2. Barrier Methods: Condoms, diaphragms, and cervical caps are examples of barrier methods that physically prevent sperm from reaching the egg.

3. Long-Acting Reversible Contraceptives (LARCs): LARCs, such as contraceptive implants and hormonal IUDs, provide long-term contraception with high effectiveness.

4. Natural Family Planning: This method involves tracking the menstrual cycle to identify fertile days and avoid intercourse during that time.

5. Permanent Methods: Sterilization procedures like tubal ligation (for women) and vasectomy (for men) offer permanent contraception.

Choosing the right contraception method involves considering factors like effectiveness, convenience, side effects, and personal preferences. Open communication with a healthcare provider is essential to make informed decisions.

Family Planning and Timing of Pregnancy:

Family planning goes beyond contraception; it includes decisions about when and how to start or expand a family. Factors such as financial stability, career goals, and personal readiness play a role in family planning. Timely discussions with a partner and healthcare provider can help individuals and couples make informed choices about the timing of pregnancy.

Common Gynecological Conditions

Understanding Gynecological Conditions:

During the reproductive years, women may encounter various gynecological conditions that can affect their reproductive health. Some common conditions include:

1. Menstrual Disorders: Conditions like heavy menstrual bleeding (menorrhagia), irregular periods (oligomenorrhea), and absence of menstruation (amenorrhea) can disrupt the menstrual cycle.

2. Polycystic Ovary Syndrome (PCOS): PCOS is a hormonal disorder that can cause irregular periods, ovarian cysts, and fertility issues.

3. Endometriosis: Endometriosis is a condition where tissue similar to the uterine lining grows outside the uterus, often causing pain and fertility problems.

4. Fibroids: Uterine fibroids are noncancerous growths in the uterus that can lead to heavy periods, pelvic pain, and fertility issues.

5. Sexually Transmitted Infections (STIs): STIs like chlamydia and gonorrhea can lead to pelvic inflammatory disease (PID), which can cause fertility problems if left untreated.

Understanding the symptoms, risk factors and treatment options for these conditions is crucial for maintaining reproductive health. Early diagnosis and management can significantly impact outcomes.

<u>Fertility and Preconception Care</u>

Fertility and Age:

Fertility is a central concern for many women during their reproductive years. It's important to understand that fertility declines with age. While women are born with a fixed number of eggs, their quantity and quality decrease over time. By age 35, fertility starts to decline more rapidly, making it harder to conceive. Knowledge of fertility trends can help individuals make informed decisions about when to start or expand their families.

Preconception Care:

Preconception care is a proactive approach to optimizing reproductive health before pregnancy. It involves:

1. Healthy Lifestyle: Adopting a healthy lifestyle that includes a balanced diet, regular exercise, and avoiding smoking and excessive alcohol consumption.

2. Managing Chronic Conditions: Addressing chronic health conditions like diabetes and hypertension to ensure they are well-controlled before conception.

3. Folic Acid Supplementation: Taking folic acid supplements before and during early pregnancy to reduce the risk of neural tube defects in the developing fetus.

4. Vaccinations: Ensuring vaccinations are up to date, including rubella and varicella vaccines, which can pose risks during pregnancy.

5. Medication Review: Consult with a healthcare provider to review and adjust medications that may be contraindicated during pregnancy.

Myths vs. Facts: Debunking Reproductive Myths

The reproductive years often come with a slew of myths and misconceptions. It's essential to debunk these myths with accurate information:

Myth 1: You can't get pregnant while breastfeeding

Fact: While breastfeeding can suppress ovulation, it's not a reliable contraceptive method. Women can still ovulate and become pregnant while breastfeeding.

Myth 2: Birth control methods always lead to infertility.

Fact: Most modern birth control methods are reversible, and fertility typically returns once the method is discontinued. However, individual responses can vary.

Myth 3: You can't get pregnant if you have irregular periods.

Fact: Irregular periods can make it challenging to predict ovulation, but it doesn't mean you can't conceive. Women with irregular cycles can still get pregnant.

Myth 4: You can't get pregnant during your period.

Fact: While the likelihood is lower, it's still possible to get pregnant during your period if you have short cycles or extended bleeding.

Nutrition and Exercise for Reproductive Health

Nutrition and exercise are foundational pillars of reproductive health during the reproductive years. A well-balanced diet and regular physical activity offer numerous benefits:

<u>Nutrition:</u>

1. Folate and Iron: Adequate folate intake is crucial for preventing neural tube defects in early pregnancy. Iron is essential to prevent anemia, especially during menstruation.

2. Calcium and Vitamin D: These nutrients support bone health, which is vital throughout a woman's life. Adequate intake is particularly important during the reproductive years.

3. Omega-3 Fatty Acids: Omega-3s support heart health and may have benefits for fertility. Fatty fish, flaxseeds, and walnuts are good sources.

4. Antioxidants: Antioxidants like vitamins C and E can help protect reproductive cells from oxidative damage.

5. Hydration: Staying well-hydrated is essential for overall health, including reproductive health.

<u>Exercise:</u>

1. Weight Management: Regular exercise helps maintain a healthy weight, which is linked to improved fertility and reduced risk of gestational diabetes during pregnancy.

2. Stress Reduction: Physical activity is an effective stress reliever, which is crucial for emotional well-being and reproductive health.

3. Hormonal Balance: Exercise can help regulate hormone levels, potentially improving menstrual regularity.

4. Bone Health: Weight-bearing exercises support bone health, reducing the risk of osteoporosis in later life.

5. Pelvic Floor Strength: Pelvic floor exercises can be beneficial for pelvic health, especially during and after pregnancy.

It's important to note that extreme exercise or excessive dieting can have negative effects on reproductive health. Striking a balance between a healthy lifestyle and excessive restrictions is key.

Chapter 3 delves into the crucial period of the reproductive years, offering comprehensive insights into reproductive health. From understanding the menstrual cycle and contraception to addressing common gynecological conditions, optimizing fertility and preconception care, and debunking myths, this chapter equips women with knowledge to navigate this significant phase. Nutrition and exercise emerge as essential components of reproductive health, reinforcing the importance of a holistic approach to well-being. By arming women with accurate information and resources, this chapter empowers them to make informed decisions and embrace their reproductive health during these vital years of life.

Chapter 4: Pregnancy and Motherhood

The journey through "Nurturing Generations: A Guide to Women's Reproductive Health" brings us to a chapter of profound significance: Pregnancy and Motherhood. This chapter explores the transformative journey of conceiving, carrying, and nurturing a child, providing a comprehensive understanding of the physical, emotional, and practical aspects that define this remarkable stage of a woman's life.

Preparing for Pregnancy

The decision to embark on the path of parenthood is a momentous one. Preparing for pregnancy involves both physical and emotional considerations:

* Health Assessment: Before conception, it's essential to undergo a health assessment. This includes reviewing medical history, addressing chronic conditions, and ensuring vaccinations are up to date.

* Folic Acid and Prenatal Vitamins: The intake of folic acid and prenatal vitamins is crucial to reduce the risk of birth defects and support the health of both mother and baby.

* Lifestyle Adjustments: Preparing for pregnancy often entails making lifestyle changes. This includes adopting a balanced diet, maintaining a healthy weight, quitting smoking, limiting alcohol consumption, and avoiding exposure to harmful substances.

* Understanding Ovulation: Understanding ovulation and tracking the menstrual cycle can help increase the chances of conception.

Pregnancy Wellness

Pregnancy is a profound and transformative journey, both physically and emotionally. Ensuring the well-being of both mother and baby is paramount:

* Prenatal Care: Regular prenatal check-ups with a healthcare provider are essential to monitor the progress of pregnancy, address any issues, and ensure optimal health for both mother and baby.

* Nutrition: A balanced diet rich in essential nutrients is vital during pregnancy. Adequate intake of folic acid, iron, calcium, and other nutrients is essential for the developing fetus.

* Exercise: Staying physically active during pregnancy offers numerous benefits, including improved mood, reduced discomfort, and enhanced stamina for labor.

* Emotional Support: Pregnancy can bring about a range of emotions. Emotional support, whether from a partner, family, or a healthcare provider, is crucial for managing stress and maintaining mental well-being.

* Common Pregnancy Symptoms: Understanding and managing common pregnancy symptoms such as nausea, fatigue, and back pain can greatly enhance comfort during pregnancy.

<u>Labor and Delivery</u>

The culmination of pregnancy is the labor and delivery process, a momentous event in a woman's life:

* Stages of Labor: Labor typically consists of three stages: the onset of contractions and dilation of the cervix, the birth of the baby, and the delivery of the placenta.

* Pain Management: There are various pain management options available during labor, including epidurals, pain-

relieving medications, and natural techniques like breathing exercises and massage.

* Childbirth Education: Childbirth education classes prepare expectant parents for labor and delivery. These classes cover topics like the stages of labor, pain management, and coping strategies.

* Birth Plans: Many expectant mothers create birth plans, outlining their preferences for labor and delivery. These plans can help ensure a more personalized birthing experience.

Postpartum Care

The period following childbirth, known as the postpartum period, is a time of adjustment and recovery:

* Physical Recovery: The body goes through significant changes during childbirth. Proper postpartum care includes monitoring physical healing, managing discomfort, and addressing any complications.

* Emotional Well-being: Postpartum emotional well-being is equally important. Some mothers experience the "baby

blues" or more severe postpartum depression. Recognizing and seeking help for emotional challenges is essential.

* Breastfeeding Support: For mothers who choose to breastfeed, support and guidance in establishing and maintaining breastfeeding is crucial. Lactation consultants and support groups can provide valuable assistance.

* Newborn Care: Learning to care for a newborn includes aspects like feeding, diapering, soothing techniques, and ensuring the baby's safety and well-being.

Breastfeeding and Infant Care

Breastfeeding is a vital aspect of infant care, offering numerous benefits for both mother and baby:

* Breastfeeding Benefits: Breast milk provides essential nutrients and antibodies to protect the baby from infections. It also promotes bonding between mother and child.

* Breastfeeding Techniques: Proper latching, positioning, and nursing frequency are essential aspects of successful breastfeeding.

* Formula Feeding: For mothers who choose not to breastfeed or encounter difficulties, formula feeding is a valid option. Choosing the right formula and ensuring proper sterilization and preparation are crucial.

* Infant Care: Caring for a newborn involves a range of activities, from diaper changes to baby-proofing the home. Learning to recognize signs of illness or distress is vital for a parent's peace of mind.

Myths vs. Facts: Separating Truth from Fiction

Pregnancy and motherhood often come with a multitude of myths and misconceptions. It's imperative to dispel these myths with accurate information:

Myth 1: You should eat for two during pregnancy:

Fact: While calorie needs increase during pregnancy, eating for two is a misconception. Focus on quality, nutrient-dense foods rather than quantity.

Myth 2: You can't exercise during pregnancy:

Fact: Exercise is encouraged during pregnancy, with modifications as needed. It can improve mood, reduce discomfort, and promote a healthy pregnancy.

Myth 3: Breastfeeding is always easy and comes naturally:

Fact: While breastfeeding is natural, it can be challenging. Many mothers benefit from lactation support and guidance.

Myth 4: A postpartum belly should bounce back immediately:

Fact: It's normal for the postpartum belly to take time to shrink. The body undergoes significant changes during pregnancy, and recovery varies among individuals.

Myth 5: Postpartum depression is rare and only affects a small percentage of women.

Fact: Postpartum depression is more common than many realize, affecting around 1 in 7 women. It's essential to seek help if experiencing symptoms.

Chapter 4 delves into the transformative journey of pregnancy and motherhood. It covers essential aspects of preparing for pregnancy, maintaining wellness during pregnancy, the labor and delivery process, postpartum care, breastfeeding, and infant care. Additionally, it dispels common myths surrounding pregnancy and motherhood, providing women with accurate information to navigate this profound stage of their reproductive journey with confidence and knowledge.

Chapter 5: Perimenopause and Menopause

In the fifth chapter of "Nurturing Generations: A Guide to Women's Reproductive Health," we delve into a phase that often carries significant physical and emotional changes for women: Perimenopause and Menopause. This chapter aims to provide a comprehensive understanding of these transitions, offering insights into recognizing their onset, managing associated symptoms, and nurturing holistic well-being.

<u>Recognizing Perimenopause</u>

Perimenopause is the transitional phase leading up to menopause. It typically begins in a woman's 40s but can start earlier or later. It's marked by a gradual decline in ovarian function, leading to fluctuating hormone levels.

<u>Common Perimenopausal Signs:</u>

Recognizing perimenopause involves understanding common signs and symptoms:

1. Irregular Periods: Menstrual cycles may become irregular, with changes in flow and duration.

2. Hot Flashes: Sudden and intense feelings of warmth, often accompanied by sweating and rapid heartbeat.

3. Night Sweats: Hot flashes that occur during sleep, leading to disrupted sleep patterns.

4. Vaginal Changes: Thinning and drying of vaginal tissues, leading to discomfort and potential pain during intercourse.

5. Mood Swings: Fluctuations in estrogen levels can affect mood, leading to irritability and emotional swings.

Managing Symptoms

Approaches to Managing Perimenopausal Symptoms:

Managing perimenopausal symptoms involves a multi-faceted approach:

1. Hormone Therapy: For some women, hormone therapy (HRT) can alleviate symptoms by replacing declining hormones. It should be discussed with a healthcare provider, considering individual health risks and benefits.

2. Lifestyle Changes: Healthy lifestyle choices, including regular exercise, a balanced diet, stress management, and adequate sleep, can help reduce symptoms.

3. Vaginal Lubricants and Moisturizers: For vaginal dryness and discomfort, over-the-counter lubricants and prescription moisturizers can provide relief.

4. Phytoestrogens: Some women find relief from symptoms by consuming foods rich in phytoestrogens, like soy products and flaxseeds.

5. Behavioral Therapies: Cognitive-behavioral therapy and mindfulness techniques can help manage mood swings and emotional symptoms.

Maintaining Bone Health

The Impact of Declining Estrogen on Bone Health:

The hormonal changes associated with perimenopause and menopause can impact bone health. Estrogen plays a significant role in maintaining bone density. As estrogen levels decline, women are at an increased risk of osteoporosis, a condition characterized by weakened and brittle bones.

<u>Maintaining Bone Health</u>:

To protect bone health during perimenopause and beyond, consider the following:

1. Calcium and Vitamin D: Adequate calcium intake and vitamin D supplementation are essential for bone health.

2. Weight-Bearing Exercise: Engaging in weight-bearing exercises like walking, jogging, or resistance training can help maintain bone density.

3. Avoiding Smoking and Excessive Alcohol: Smoking and excessive alcohol consumption can negatively impact bone health.

4. Bone Density Testing: For women at higher risk of osteoporosis, bone density testing may be recommended.

<u>The Emotional Landscape of Perimenopause and Menopause:</u>

Perimenopause and menopause can bring about emotional and mental challenges. Hormonal fluctuations can contribute to mood swings, irritability, and increased vulnerability to conditions like anxiety and depression.

Strategies for Emotional Well-being:

Caring for emotional well-being during perimenopause and menopause involves:

1. Open Communication: Discussing emotional changes with loved ones and healthcare providers can provide support and guidance.

2. Supportive Social Network: Maintaining strong social connections can buffer against feelings of isolation and loneliness.

3. Stress Management: Techniques like mindfulness, relaxation exercises, and yoga can help manage stress.

4. Professional Help: Seeking therapy or counseling can be beneficial for managing mood disorders or emotional distress.

Myths vs. Facts: Clarifying Misunderstandings

Perimenopause and menopause are often shrouded in myths and misconceptions. Clarifying these misunderstandings is essential for informed decision-making:

Myth 1: All women experience severe symptoms during perimenopause and menopause.

Fact: While many women do experience symptoms, their severity and duration can vary widely. Some women may have mild symptoms, while others may have more severe challenges.

Myth 2: Hormone therapy (HRT) is the only way to manage menopausal symptoms.

Fact: Hormone therapy is one option, but there are various approaches to symptom management, including lifestyle changes, non-hormonal medications, and complementary therapies.

Myth 3: Menopause signifies the end of a woman's sexual life.

Fact: While changes in hormone levels can impact sexual function, many women continue to enjoy fulfilling sexual lives during and after menopause. Open communication with a partner and healthcare provider can help address any challenges.

Myth 4: Osteoporosis is an inevitable part of aging for women

Fact: Osteoporosis can be prevented or managed with lifestyle modifications, including a healthy diet, weight-bearing exercise, and adequate calcium and vitamin D intake.

Myth 5: Emotional changes during menopause are purely hormonal and cannot be managed.

Fact: Emotional changes during menopause can be managed through various strategies, including therapy, stress management, and social support.

In summary, Chapter 5 offers comprehensive insights into perimenopause and menopause, addressing the recognition of these phases, management of associated symptoms, the importance of bone health, strategies for emotional and mental well-being, and the clarification of common myths and misconceptions. By equipping women with knowledge and support, this chapter empowers them to navigate perimenopause and menopause with resilience, confidence, and holistic well-being.

Chapter 6: Golden Years: Reproductive Health in Later Life

In this chapter, we explore a phase of life often celebrated for wisdom and experience: the Golden Years. This chapter provides valuable insights into the unique considerations of reproductive health as women age, addressing aging's impact on reproductive health, pelvic health and incontinence, maintaining intimacy, and postmenopausal health.

Aging and Reproductive Health

Reproductive Health Transitions:

As women age, their reproductive health undergoes significant transitions. Menopause, the cessation of menstruation, typically occurs between the ages of 45 and 55. This marks the end of a woman's reproductive years, as ovaries no longer release eggs, and hormone levels, especially estrogen, decline.

Impacts on Reproductive Health:

Aging has several effects on reproductive health:

1. Menopause Symptoms: Many women experience symptoms like hot flashes, night sweats, and vaginal dryness during menopause.

2. Bone Health: Declining estrogen levels increase the risk of osteoporosis, a condition characterized by brittle bones.

3. Cardiovascular Health: Changes in hormones can affect heart health, emphasizing the importance of cardiovascular care.

4. Sexual Health: Vaginal dryness and changes in sexual desire may impact sexual health.

5. Cancer Risk: Age is a significant risk factor for certain cancers, including breast and ovarian cancer.

Pelvic Health and Incontinence

Pelvic Health in Later Life:

Maintaining pelvic health is crucial as women age. The pelvic floor muscles, which support the bladder, uterus, and rectum, can weaken over time. This may lead to issues like urinary incontinence, fecal incontinence, or pelvic organ prolapse.

Incontinence Types and Management:

Understanding incontinence types and management strategies is essential:

1. Stress Incontinence: This occurs during activities that put pressure on the bladder, such as laughing, sneezing, or lifting. Pelvic floor exercises (Kegels) and lifestyle changes can help manage stress incontinence.

2. Urge Incontinence: Characterized by a sudden and strong urge to urinate, often leading to leakage. Behavioral therapies, medications, and bladder training can assist with urge incontinence.

3. Mixed Incontinence: A combination of stress and urge incontinence. Treatment may involve a combination of approaches.

4. Fecal Incontinence: This condition involves the inability to control bowel movements. Dietary adjustments, medication, and pelvic floor exercises can aid in management.

<u>Maintaining Intimacy</u>

Maintaining Sexual Intimacy:

Physical and emotional intimacy remain essential aspects of a fulfilling life during the Golden Years. Addressing changes in sexual health can help maintain intimacy:

1. Communication: Open and honest communication with a partner about desires, challenges, and preferences is crucial.

2. Vaginal Dryness: Lubricants and moisturizers can alleviate vaginal dryness and discomfort.

3. Hormone Therapy: For some women, hormone therapy may improve sexual function.

4. Emotional Connection: Emotional intimacy, trust, and affection are integral to sexual satisfaction.

<u>Postmenopausal Health</u>

Postmenopausal Health Considerations:

Postmenopausal health encompasses a range of considerations:

1. Bone Health: Osteoporosis risk remains, and maintaining bone density through diet, exercise, and, if necessary, medication is crucial.

2. Cardiovascular Health: As heart disease risk increases with age, lifestyle measures like a heart-healthy diet and regular exercise are essential.

3. Breast Health: Regular breast health screenings, including mammograms, remain important.

4. Screening for Other Cancers: Appropriate cancer screenings, such as pap smears and colorectal cancer screenings, should continue based on individual risk factors and healthcare provider recommendations.

5. Pelvic Health: Maintaining pelvic floor strength through exercises and addressing any incontinence issues is vital.

6. Mental Health: Addressing mental health, including potential mood disorders, depression, and cognitive changes, is important.

<u>Holistic Well-being in the Golden Years</u>

Aging can be a fulfilling and vibrant phase of life. Holistic well-being in the Golden Years involves:

1. Lifestyle Choices: Continuing to make healthy choices regarding diet, exercise, and stress management.

2. Regular Check-ups: Routine medical check-ups and screenings to monitor and manage health conditions.

3. Social Engagement: Maintaining social connections and a strong support system.

4. Mental Stimulation: Engaging in activities that challenge the mind and promote cognitive health.

5. Embracing Change: Embracing the changes that come with aging while seeking opportunities for growth and enrichment.

 Chapter 6 of addresses the unique considerations of reproductive health in the Golden Years. Aging impacts various aspects of health, including menopause, pelvic health, intimacy, and overall well-being. By understanding these changes and adopting strategies to maintain health and vitality, women can navigate the Golden Years with grace, resilience, and an enduring commitment to their reproductive well-being.

Chapter 7: Holistic Approaches to Reproductive Wellness

In this chapter, we explore a holistic perspective on reproductive wellness. This chapter is dedicated to understanding the interconnectedness of nutrition, exercise, the mind-body connection, herbal remedies, natural treatments, stress management, and self-care in fostering reproductive well-being.

Nutrition and Dietary Choices

The Power of Nutrition:

Nutrition plays a fundamental role in reproductive health. The foods we consume provide essential nutrients that support hormonal balance, fertility, and overall well-being. Key aspects of nutrition include:

1. Balanced Diet: A diet rich in fruits, vegetables, whole grains, lean proteins, and healthy fats provides a wide range of nutrients necessary for reproductive health.

2. Folic Acid: Folic acid is crucial for preventing birth defects. It's recommended for women planning to conceive and during pregnancy.

3. Iron: Iron is essential for maintaining healthy blood and preventing anemia, a condition that can affect fertility and pregnancy.

4. Calcium and Vitamin D: Adequate intake of calcium and vitamin D supports bone health, which is crucial for pregnancy and overall wellness.

5. Antioxidants: Antioxidants found in foods like berries, nuts, and leafy greens help protect reproductive cells from oxidative stress.

6. Omega-3 Fatty Acids: These fats, found in fish, flaxseeds, and walnuts, support hormonal balance and may improve fertility.

<u>Exercise and Physical Activity</u>

Benefits of Physical Activity:

Regular exercise offers numerous benefits for reproductive health:

1. Hormonal Balance: Exercise helps regulate hormonal levels, potentially improving menstrual regularity and fertility.

2. Weight Management: Maintaining a healthy weight is essential for reproductive wellness. Exercise assists in weight management.

3. Stress Reduction: Physical activity is a powerful stress reducer, promoting emotional well-being.

4. Bone Health: Weight-bearing exercises strengthen bones, reducing the risk of osteoporosis.

5. Cardiovascular Health: Exercise supports heart health, vital for a healthy pregnancy.

6. Improved Circulation: Good circulation is essential for reproductive organs and fertility.

Mind-Body Connection

Embracing Mind-Body Wellness:

The mind-body connection acknowledges the profound impact of mental and emotional well-being on reproductive health:

1. Stress Reduction: Chronic stress can affect fertility and menstrual regularity. Mindfulness, meditation, and relaxation techniques help manage stress.

2. Emotional Health: Addressing emotional challenges, such as anxiety or depression, is essential for overall well-being.

3. Fertility Awareness: Techniques like the Fertility Awareness Method involve tracking menstrual cycles and recognizing fertile days, aiding in family planning.

4. Psychological Support: Therapy or counseling can provide valuable support for managing emotional aspects of reproductive health.

<u>Herbal Remedies and Natural Treatments</u>

Herbal and Natural Approaches:

Herbal remedies and natural treatments have been used for centuries to address reproductive health concerns. Key considerations include:

1. Herbal Supplements: Some herbs, like chasteberry and red clover, are believed to support hormonal balance and menstrual regularity.

2. **Acupuncture: Traditional Chinese medicine, including acupuncture, is sometimes used to enhance fertility and address reproductive issues.

3. Aromatherapy: Essential oils can be used for relaxation and stress reduction, supporting emotional well-being.

4. Natural Family Planning: Methods like cervical mucus monitoring and basal body temperature tracking can aid in natural family planning.

5. Homeopathy: Homeopathic remedies are used by some individuals to address various reproductive health concerns.

Stress Management and Self-care

Prioritizing Stress Management:

Stress can profoundly impact reproductive health. Stress management and self-care strategies are essential:

1. Self-care Rituals: Activities like reading, spending time in nature, or engaging in hobbies promote relaxation and self-nurturing.

2. Time Management: Effective time management helps reduce stress and provides opportunities for self-care.

3. Sleep Hygiene: Quality sleep is essential for hormonal balance and overall wellness.

4. Yoga and Meditation: These practices enhance relaxation, reduce stress, and promote emotional balance.

5. Breathing Exercises: Deep breathing techniques can be used throughout the day to manage stress and promote calm.

6. Professional Support: Seeking support from a therapist or counselor can be invaluable for managing stress and emotional challenges.

In summary, Chapter 7 explores holistic approaches to reproductive wellness. Nutrition, exercise, the mind-body connection, herbal remedies, natural treatments, stress management, and self-care all play integral roles in promoting reproductive health and overall well-being. By recognizing the interplay between these elements and adopting a holistic approach, women can nurture their reproductive health and embrace a vibrant, balanced, and fulfilling life.

Chapter 8: Accessible Healthcare for All

In the final chapter of "Nurturing Generations: A Guide to Women's Reproductive Health," we delve into the vital topic of accessible healthcare for all. This chapter addresses healthcare rights and advocacy, finding trusted healthcare providers, exploring affordable healthcare options, utilizing telehealth and online resources, and dispelling common myths to empower women in navigating the complex world of healthcare.

<u>Healthcare Rights and Advocacy</u>

Understanding Healthcare Rights:

Every individual possesses inherent healthcare rights that ensure equitable access to medical services and protection against discrimination. Key aspects of healthcare rights include:

1. Right to Information: Patients have the right to receive clear and understandable information about their medical condition, treatment options, and potential risks.

2. Informed Consent: Informed consent is a fundamental right, ensuring that patients are informed about and agree to medical procedures and treatments.

3. Privacy and Confidentiality: Medical information must be kept confidential, respecting the patient's right to privacy.

4. Non-Discrimination: Healthcare providers are obligated to treat all patients equally, regardless of race, gender, age, or other characteristics.

5. Access to Medical Records: Patients have the right to access their medical records and request amendments or corrections.

6. Complaints and Appeals: Patients can voice concerns or complaints about their healthcare and seek resolution.

Healthcare Advocacy:

Advocacy is essential to ensure that healthcare rights are upheld. Patients and advocacy organizations play a crucial role in raising awareness of healthcare disparities, fighting discrimination, and promoting equitable access to healthcare services.

<u>Finding a Trusted Healthcare Provider</u>

Choosing a Healthcare Provider:

Selecting a healthcare provider is a pivotal decision that influences the quality of care received. Key considerations include:

1. Credentials and Experience: Verify the qualifications, certifications, and experience of healthcare providers to ensure they meet your specific needs.

2. Referrals and Recommendations: Seek referrals from trusted sources, such as friends, family, or primary care physicians.

3. Insurance Coverage: Verify that the provider accepts your health insurance plan to minimize out-of-pocket expenses.

4. Location and Accessibility: Consider the location of the healthcare facility and its accessibility, particularly if you have mobility challenges.

5. Communication and Trust: Effective communication and trust between the patient and provider are essential for quality care.

<u>Affordable Healthcare Options</u>

Access to Affordable Healthcare:

Affordable healthcare is a fundamental right. Exploring healthcare options that fit one's financial situation is crucial:

1. Health Insurance: Health insurance plans, whether private or government-funded, provide coverage for medical expenses. Understanding your insurance plan's coverage and costs is essential.

2. Medicaid and Medicare: These government programs provide healthcare coverage to eligible individuals, particularly those with low incomes or who are elderly.

3. Community Clinics: Federally qualified health centers and community clinics offer affordable or sliding-scale fee services to underserved populations.

4. Prescription Assistance Programs: Many pharmaceutical companies offer programs to help individuals afford necessary medications.

5. Health Savings Accounts (HSAs) and Flexible Spending Accounts (FSAs) : These financial tools can assist in saving for medical expenses and provide tax benefits.

<u>Telehealth and Online Resources</u>

The Rise of Telehealth:

Telehealth, or the use of technology to provide healthcare services remotely, has become increasingly prevalent. Its benefits include:

1. Convenience: Telehealth allows patients to access healthcare from the comfort of their homes, reducing travel time and costs.

2. Accessibility: It extends healthcare services to individuals in remote or underserved areas.

3. Specialized Consultations: Patients can access specialized care and consultations from experts regardless of geographical location.

4. Timely Care: Telehealth can expedite the diagnosis and treatment of medical issues, improving health outcomes.

5. Mental Health Services: Teletherapy and online resources are valuable for mental health support and counseling.

Myths vs. Facts: Navigating Healthcare Realities

Dispelling Common Healthcare Myths:

Myth 1: Only wealthy individuals can afford quality healthcare.

Fact: Affordable healthcare options, including insurance plans, government programs, and community clinics, ensure that quality care is accessible to individuals across income levels.

Myth 2: Health insurance guarantees complete coverage, and there are no out-of-pocket costs.

Fact: Most health insurance plans involve some out-of-pocket costs, including copayments, deductibles, and coinsurance. Understanding your plan is crucial to managing costs.

Myth 3: Telehealth is not as effective as in-person healthcare.

Fact: Telehealth has proven to be effective for a wide range of medical services, providing convenient and timely care while maintaining quality.

Myth 4: Healthcare providers always know best, and patients should not question their recommendations.

Fact: Patients have the right to participate in their healthcare decisions, ask questions, and seek second opinions when needed. Effective communication between patient and provider is essential.

Myth 5: Healthcare disparities no longer exist in modern society.

Fact: Healthcare disparities persist, affecting access to care and health outcomes among different demographic groups.

Addressing disparities through policy changes and advocacy remains crucial.

In summary, Chapter 8 of "Nurturing Generations: A Guide to Women's Reproductive Health" emphasizes the importance of accessible healthcare for all. It explores healthcare rights and advocacy, choosing trusted providers, affordable healthcare options, the rise of telehealth, and dispelling common myths. By empowering women with knowledge and resources, this chapter equips them to navigate the healthcare system with confidence, ensuring that their reproductive health and overall well-being are prioritized and protected.

Chapter 9: Empowering Women Globally

In this Chapter, we extend our focus beyond individual well-being to address the critical imperative of empowering women globally. This chapter is dedicated to understanding the state of reproductive health worldwide, dispelling myths that span cultures and nations, identifying the challenges women face globally, exploring solutions to these challenges, and highlighting the vital role of support and international organizations in advancing women's reproductive rights and well-being on a global scale.

Reproductive Health Worldwide

The Global Reproductive Health Landscape:

Reproductive health is a universal concern, impacting women of all ages, backgrounds, and geographic locations. A comprehensive understanding of global reproductive health involves recognizing common issues and variations across regions:

1. Fertility Rates: Fertility rates vary worldwide, influenced by cultural norms, economic factors, and access to contraception and family planning.

2. Maternal Mortality: Maternal mortality rates reflect disparities in healthcare access and quality, with higher rates in developing countries.

3. Contraception Access: Availability and affordability of contraception differ across nations, affecting family planning choices and reproductive health outcomes.

4. Unsafe Abortion: In regions with restrictive abortion laws, women often resort to unsafe abortion methods, resulting in significant health risks.

5. Adolescent Reproductive Health: Young girls and adolescents may face unique challenges in accessing reproductive healthcare and information.

6. Gender-Based Violence: Gender-based violence, including female genital mutilation and child marriage, remains a pervasive issue in some parts of the world, profoundly impacting reproductive health.

Myths vs. Facts: Bridging Cultural and Global Myths

Myth 1: Women don't need reproductive health education.

Fact: Access to accurate reproductive health information is essential for informed decisions about contraception, pregnancy, and overall well-being.

Myth 2: Family planning is a Western concept and not suitable for all cultures.

Fact: Family planning is a universal need, and approaches should be culturally sensitive and tailored to individual values and beliefs.

Myth 3: Contraception leads to infertility.

Fact: The majority of contraception methods do not impact future fertility. Temporary infertility may occur immediately after discontinuation of certain methods.

Myth 4: Abortion is always dangerous and harmful to women's health.

Fact: Safe, legal, and medically supervised abortion is a critical reproductive healthcare option that can be performed without harm to women's health.

Myth 5: Adolescent sexuality should not be discussed openly.

Fact: Open and age-appropriate discussions about adolescent sexuality are essential for informed choices and preventing unintended pregnancies and STIs.

<u>Challenges and Solutions</u>

Global Challenges in Reproductive Health:

Numerous challenges persist in promoting reproductive health globally, including:

1. Limited Access to Healthcare: Many women lack access to essential reproductive healthcare services, including prenatal care, safe childbirth, and family planning.

2. Cultural and Societal Norms: Cultural practices and societal norms can restrict women's autonomy in making reproductive health decisions.

3. Education Gaps: Lack of comprehensive sexual education and information contributes to misinformation and poor reproductive health outcomes.

4. Healthcare Infrastructure: Inadequate healthcare infrastructure in some regions hinders the delivery of quality reproductive healthcare.

5. Economic Barriers: Financial constraints can limit access to contraception, maternal care, and safe abortion services.

<u>Global Solutions and Initiatives</u>:

Addressing these challenges requires a collaborative effort:

1. Comprehensive Sexual Education: Implementing comprehensive sexual education programs can equip individuals with accurate information and empower them to make informed decisions.

2. Accessible Healthcare: Expanding access to affordable, quality healthcare services, including family planning and maternal care, is essential.

3. Community Engagement: Engaging communities and local leaders in discussions about reproductive health can foster cultural sensitivity and acceptance.

4. Gender Equality: Promoting gender equality and women's empowerment are central to addressing reproductive health disparities.

5. International Partnerships: Collaborative efforts among governments, NGOs, and international organizations are crucial in advancing global reproductive health initiatives.

Support and International Organizations

The Roles of International Organizations in Reproductive Health:

1. UNFPA (United Nations Population Fund): UNFPA works to ensure that every pregnancy is wanted, every childbirth is safe, and every young person's potential Is fulfIlled.

2. WHO (World Health Organization): WHO provides evidence-based guidance on reproductive health, maternal health, and family planning.

3. Planned Parenthood: Planned Parenthood affiliates worldwide provide reproductive healthcare, education, and advocacy.

4. Marie Stopes International: This organization offers contraception and safe abortion services in various countries.

5. International Planned Parenthood Federation (IPPF): IPPF operates globally, advocating for sexual and reproductive rights and providing healthcare services.

Local Initiatives and Grassroots Efforts

Local and grassroots organizations play an essential role in addressing specific regional challenges and tailoring reproductive health solutions to local contexts.

Individual Action and Advocacy:

Individuals can contribute to global reproductive health by advocating for policy changes, supporting international organizations, and raising awareness about reproductive health issues:

1. Policy Advocacy: Individuals can advocate for policies that promote reproductive health and rights, both locally and globally. This includes supporting legislation that ensures access to comprehensive sexual education, contraception, and safe abortion services.

2. Donations and Fundraising: Supporting international organizations financially helps them continue their critical work in improving reproductive health worldwide.

3. Volunteer and Outreach: Individuals can volunteer their time and expertise to organizations involved in reproductive health initiatives, contributing to education and support efforts.

4. Raise Awareness: Raising awareness about global reproductive health issues through social media, community events, and educational campaigns helps shine a light on the challenges women face and the importance of reproductive rights.

5. Educate Yourself: Staying informed about global reproductive health issues and staying up-to-date with current research and developments is essential to be an effective advocate.

In summary, Chapter 9 emphasizes the importance of empowering women globally in matters of reproductive health. It explores the global landscape of reproductive health, dispels cross-cultural myths, identifies challenges and solutions, and highlights the crucial role of support and international organizations. By recognizing the shared challenges women face and collaborating on solutions, individuals, organizations, and governments can work together to ensure that every woman, regardless of her location or background, has the opportunity to enjoy reproductive health and rights as a fundamental aspect of her well-being.

Conclusion

As we come to the close of "**Nurturing Generations: A Guide to Women's Reproductive Health**," we reflect on the incredible journey we've undertaken together. This book has been a comprehensive exploration of the myriad facets of women's reproductive health, from the earliest stages of life to the golden years, and from the deeply personal to the global. It has been a journey of knowledge, empowerment, and inspiration.

Throughout this book, we have delved into the essential aspects of women's reproductive health. We've learned about the stages of life, from childhood and adolescence to the reproductive years, pregnancy, perimenopause, and menopause. We've explored the myths and facts that surround these stages, debunking misconceptions and shedding light on the realities. We've discussed holistic approaches to reproductive wellness, including nutrition, exercise, the mind-body connection, herbal remedies, and stress management. We've navigated the complexities of accessing healthcare and the critical importance of advocating for your rights. We've celebrated personal stories of empowerment, resilience, and success that have inspired us all.

As we conclude, remember that your reproductive health journey is a lifelong commitment to yourself. It's about embracing your body, understanding its needs, and making informed choices that empower you to lead a healthy and fulfilling life. It's about seeking knowledge, asking questions, and advocating for your rights and well-being. It's about supporting others on their journeys and fostering a community of understanding and compassion.

Your reproductive health is not just a matter of biology; it's a reflection of your strength, resilience, and capacity for growth. It's an affirmation of your worth and your right to lead a life that is both healthy and meaningful. Your journey is unique, but it's also part of a broader tapestry of shared experiences that bind us together as women.

Resources for Further Information

The journey doesn't end here. As you continue on your path of reproductive health, there are numerous resources available to support you:

1. Healthcare Providers: Your trusted healthcare provider is a valuable source of information and guidance. Don't hesitate to ask questions and seek their expertise.

2. Books and Publications: There are many books, articles, and publications dedicated to women's reproductive health. Continue to explore and educate yourself.

3. Online Communities: Joining online communities or forums can provide a platform for discussion, sharing experiences, and seeking advice from others who have walked similar paths.

4. Advocacy Groups: There are numerous advocacy groups and organizations dedicated to advancing women's reproductive rights and health. Consider becoming involved or seeking their support.

5. Mental Health Resources: If you're facing mental health challenges related to reproductive health, don't hesitate to seek professional help. Mental health support is an essential part of your overall well-being.

6. Global Initiatives: For those interested in global reproductive health issues, consider supporting or getting involved with international organizations working to make a difference.

Remember, your journey is ongoing, and there is always more to learn, explore, and achieve. Your commitment to your reproductive health is an investment in yourself and in the generations to come.

As we bid farewell to this book, may you carry its wisdom with you, and may you continue to nurture your own well-being and empower others in their reproductive health journeys. Together, we can create a world where every woman has the knowledge, resources, and support she needs to thrive.

Appendices

Appendix A: Glossary of Terms

- Amenorrhea

- Cervix

- Endometriosis

- Fertility

- Menopause

- Ovulation

- Pap Smear

- Perimenopause

- Reproductive System

- STD (Sexually Transmitted Disease)

Appendix B: Recommended Reading List

1. "Taking Charge of Your Fertility" by Toni Weschler

2. "The Vagina Bible" by Dr. Jen Gunter

3. "The Fifth Vital Sign" by Lisa Hendrickson-Jack

4. "The Hormone Cure" by Dr. Sara Gottfried

5. "Expecting Better" by Emily Oster

6. "Ina May's Guide to Childbirth" by Ina May Gaskin

7. "The Red Tent" by Anita Diamant

8. "Period Power" by Maisie Hill

9. "Taking Care of Your Down There: A Guide to Vaginal Health and Hygiene" by Dr. Jennifer Berman and Dr. Laura Berman

10. "The Womanly Art of Breastfeeding" by La Leche League International

Appendix C: Additional Resources

1. Planned Parenthood (plannedparenthood.org)

2. American Pregnancy Association (americanpregnancy.org)

3. The World Health Organization (WHO) (who.int)

4. Center for Disease Control and Prevention (CDC) (cdc.gov)

5. The International Federation of Gynecology and Obstetrics (FIGO) (figo.org)

6. International Confederation of Midwives (ICM) (internationalmidwives.org)

7. National Women's Health Network (nwhn.org)

8. Association of Reproductive Health Professionals (ARHP) (arhp.org)

9. The Global Library of Women's Medicine (GLOWM) (glowm.com)

10. National Organization for Women (NOW) (now.org)